YOUR KNOWLEDGE HAS VALUE

- We will publish your bachelor's and master's thesis, essays and papers

- Your own eBook and book - sold worldwide in all relevant shops

- Earn money with each sale

Upload your text at www.GRIN.com
and publish for free

Bibliographic information published by the German National Library:

The German National Library lists this publication in the National Bibliography; detailed bibliographic data are available on the Internet at http://dnb.dnb.de .

This book is copyright material and must not be copied, reproduced, transferred, distributed, leased, licensed or publicly performed or used in any way except as specifically permitted in writing by the publishers, as allowed under the terms and conditions under which it was purchased or as strictly permitted by applicable copyright law. Any unauthorized distribution or use of this text may be a direct infringement of the author s and publisher s rights and those responsible may be liable in law accordingly.

Imprint:

Copyright © 2016 GRIN Verlag
Print and binding: Books on Demand GmbH, Norderstedt Germany
ISBN: 9783668730359

This book at GRIN:

https://www.grin.com/document/429725

Rodney Mulelu, Marie Matee

Lived Experiences of People Living with HIV (PLHIV) and on Antiretroviral Therapy in South Africa

GRIN Verlag

GRIN - Your knowledge has value

Since its foundation in 1998, GRIN has specialized in publishing academic texts by students, college teachers and other academics as e-book and printed book. The website www.grin.com is an ideal platform for presenting term papers, final papers, scientific essays, dissertations and specialist books.

Visit us on the internet:

http://www.grin.com/

http://www.facebook.com/grincom

http://www.twitter.com/grin_com

LIVED EXPERIENCES OF PEOPLE LIVING WITH HIV (PLHIV) AND ON ANTIRETROVIRAL THERAPY IN SOUTH AFRICA.

Author: Mr. Rodney Azwinndini Mulelu (MBA, MA-HIV),
Co-Author: Ms. Marie Matee (MA-HIV)

UNIVERSITY OF SOUTH AFRICA (UNISA), PRETORIA, SOUTH AFRICA

Abstract: The researcher investigated the lived experiences of people living with the Human Immunodeficiency Virus (HIV) and who are accessing antiretroviral treatment at a public health clinic in Limpopo, South Africa. A qualitative method was used. The research findings revealed five themes: experiences, social support, knowledge, attitudes, unemployment and economic themes of the study. Factors reported influencing optimum adherence were the inability of the patients to take medication at work, laziness of the patients to collect medication, unemployment, economic hardship, poverty and lack of knowledge of employers regarding HIV/AIDS.

Key word: HIV/AIDS knowledge, HIV/AIDS attitude, People living with HIV, HIV/AIDS experiences, Adherence, Wellness clinic, antiretroviral treatment

1. INTRODUCTION 3
2. THE RESEARCH PROBLEM 3
3. AIM OF THE STUDY 3
4. OBJECTIVES OF THE STUDY 3
5. RESEARCH DESIGN 4
6. SAMPLING STRATEGIES 4
   6.1. Sampling strategy 4
7. DATA GENERATION STRATEGIES 4
   7.1. Face-to-face interviews 5
8. ACCESS NEGOTIATION AND ETHICAL CONSIDERATIONS 5
   8.1. Informed consent 5
   8.2. Voluntary participation 5
   8.3. Confidentiality 5
9. DATA ANALYSIS 6
   9.1. Data analysis strategies for the study 6
10. LIVED EXPERIENCES OF PLHIV AND ON ANTIRETROVIRAL TREATMENT 6
    10.1. Knowledge regarding Antiretroviral treatment 6
    10.2. Attitudes to Antiretroviral treatment 7
    10.3. Experiences of people living with HIV on Antiretroviral treatment 8
11. DISCUSSION OF THE FINDINGS 8
    11.1. Introduction 8
    11.2. Sumary of Findings According to the Objectives 8
      11.2.1. Objective 1: Knowledge of People Living with HIV Towards Antiretroviral Treatment 8
      11.2.2. Objective 2: Attitudes of People Living with HIV Regarding Antiretroviral Treatment 9
      11.2.3. Objective 3: Experiences of People Living With HIV Towards Antiretroviral Treatment 9
      11.2.4. Objective 4: Economic Factors that Support People Living with HIV 10
12. CONCLUSION 10
13. REFERENCES 11

1. INTRODUCTION

Despite advances in the prevention strategies the HIV and AIDS pandemic is still one of the most challenging health issues that South Africa has ever had to deal with post apartheid era. The Antiretroviral therapy programme is one of the biggest in the world with more than 3.5 million people accessing HIV treatment and more than 7 million people living with the disease[1]. Furthermore, HIV and AIDS pose a serious threat to the social and economic development of the country. In addition, South Africa has only 0.7% of the world population but is carrying 17% of the HIV and AIDS burden of the world. Adherence to ARV therapy is essential to maintaining long-term health benefits, and avoiding the development of viral resistance [1].

However, there is a need for strong support systems for PLHIV and that systems should be established within the facilities that render comprehensive care management and treatment of PLHIV, including ART [2]. Counselors trained on the ART programme could facilitate the establishment of support groups for people taking ART as their chronic medication and to reinforced community-based structures. Furthermore, People living with HIV and on ART have to be encouraged to identify social support structures in their communities and to disclose their HIV sero-status, as these factors directly impact on the success of an ART programme [2].

2. THE RESEARCH PROBLEM

Antiretroviral medication regimes for HIV infection are complex and inconvenient to PLHIV. They often produce side-effects and must be taken for long periods [3]. The minimum level of adherence required for ARVs to work efficiently is 95%. Furthermore, important socio-economic predictors of ART adherence include transport and access to health service. It is important for the patients to take seriously the issues of adherence and commit to their treatment for the ART programme to be a success [4]. The failure to adhere to treatment satisfactorily leads to complications or progression of varied diseases [5]. Barriers to adherence included fear of disclosure, forgetfulness, health illiteracy, financial constraints and patients being away from their medications [6].

3. AIM OF THE STUDY

The aim of this study was to assess the knowledge, attitudes and experiences of people living with HIV and who are on antiretroviral treatment (ART) at a public health clinic in Limpopo, South Africa.

4. OBJECTIVES OF THE STUDY

The following objectives were formulated to guide this study. The researcher wanted to:

- Assess the knowledge that people living with HIV have on ART.
- Identify attitudes of people living with HIV towards ART.
- Discover the experiences of people living with HIV and on ART.

5. RESEARCH DESIGN

The research was conducted using the qualitative enquiry method to collect data. Qualitative researchers exemplify a common belief that this method can provide a deeper understanding of the social phenomenon than would be obtained from purely quantitative data [7]. The goal of the study was to evaluate the knowledge, attitudes and experiences of people living with HIV and on ART in the health facility. Given this goal, a qualitative method approach was called for.

Furthermore, qualitative design explores attitudes, behavior and experiences through such methods as open-ended, face to face interviews and focus groups. In this study, data were collected using interviews conducted with the people living with HIV who are on ART [8]. In addition, qualitative research is any data gathering technique that generates open-ended, narrative data. It tends to be exploratory and descriptive in nature and designed to develop an understanding of individuals in their natural environment [9]. In this study, the researcher interviewed participants to be able to gain an understanding of the concept being studied. Qualitative design was preferred because it gave the participants an opportunity to talk and expand more on the topic and answer open-ended questions [10]. The aim was not to generalize, but to get the understanding of the issues related to knowledge, attitude and experiences of the participants.

6. SAMPLING STRATEGIES

Sampling is defined as the selection of some units to represent the entire population from which the units were drawn. There is very little or no assumption that the sample will be representative of the larger population and as a result the findings cannot be generalized [11]. In purposive sampling, the researcher uses his/her own judgments when selecting possible participants for the study [12]. In this study, the researcher used purposive sampling strategy to select the participants.

6.1. Sampling strategy

Efficient sample size in a qualitative study is dependent on the amount, depth and richness of the data the researcher wants to gather [13]. Following the intensity sampling strategy as described by Collins, Onwuegbuzie and Jiao [14], the researcher purposely recruited participants attending the wellness clinic in the facility. The participants for the face-to-face interviews were purposefully chosen as they present themselves at the wellness clinic. On a daily basis, clients present to a dietician consulting room for dietetic services. As they present to the Dietician (researcher), the researcher had an opportunity to request them to participate in the study. Those accepted to be part of the study were interviewed and five participants accepted to participate in the interviews.

7. DATA GENERATION STRATEGIES

Since a qualitative research design was used [15], the researcher followed one data generation strategy. It is discussed in greater detail below. Data collection is defined as the precise and systematic gathering of information relevant to the research purpose, objectives and questions. The researcher was totally involved and able to interact with the participants[9].

7.1. Face-to-face interviews

Interview schedule is defined as a written list of questions, open or closed-ended, prepared for use by an interviewer, in a person to person interaction [16]. In addition, this may be face-to-face or by use of telephone or any media. The researcher used face-to-face interviews as a method of data collection.

The face-to-face interviews were approached as structured conversations based on the on a pre-arranged set of questions[16].The interview sessions were scheduled over five days in the Witpoort Hospital dietician private room in June 2013. All sessions interviews were tape-recorded and notes were taken as a back-up. The researcher commenced each interview by greeting his interviewees and thanking them for taking part in the study. Each interview took about half an hour to an hour. All interviews were conducted in Sepedi, but interviewees were also allowed to express themselves in their language of choice.

8. ACCESS NEGOTIATION AND ETHICAL CONSIDERATIONS

The researcher did not encounter any difficulties with accessing his units of observation (which were five people living with HIV who are on ART) as he had been working in this Hospital as a Dietician. In considering the ethical implications of the study, the researcher tried to remain true to the notion of this study as a critical examination of underlying social systems with the purpose of furthering human rights and social justice [17].

In addition, the provision of dietetic services to people living with HIV was regarded as a human right and those rights are being upheld in the interest of social justice. It was not difficult for the researcher to conduct the interviews as an insider of the research site, because he followed all the relevant ethical considerations in conducting social research. The basic considerations when conducting social research involve recognizing and making ethical choices, making principled decisions, ensuring confidentiality and obtaining informed consent from participants whilst maintain research integrity[18]. The basic procedural considerations that guided the data generation and data analysis steps followed in this study are discussed below.

8.1. Informed consent

The researcher provided accurate information to his participants regarding the purpose of the study and what participation entailed.

8.2. Voluntary participation

The participants in this study had the right to voluntary decide whether or not to participate. Participants also had the right to terminate their participation at any time during the study without fear of intimidation or penalties. The researcher informed all the participants about the purpose of the study and participants voluntarily participated.

8.3. Confidentiality

Interviews were conducted in a private room. Confidentiality refers to protecting and not sharing personal information of the participants without their consent [19]. In this study, the collected information, recordings, informed consent forms and other project materials were kept in a locked space at researcher's office. The information was accessible to the researcher alone. The tape recorder was password protected and only available to researcher. The researcher is planning to dispose of the raw data five years after the degree has been conferred.

9. DATA ANALYSIS

The interviews data, which was collected by means of tape recorder, was transcribed. The theoretical framework used in the research guided the conceptualization of the categories and themes in the data analysis.

9.1. Data analysis strategies for the study

In this study, data analysis will start with listening to the tape recordings numerous times. The tape recorded interviews will be transcribed and translated to English. Similar patterns were extracted from the interview transcripts. The data were coded and analyzed manually. Themes were identified. In *thematic analysis*, the researcher is predominantly interested in the emergence of themes from the collected data

10. LIVED EXPERIENCES OF PLHIV AND ON ANTIRETROVIRAL TREATMENT

The study that was conducted by Dimatteao and others looked into the model to improve adherence to antiretroviral treatment. The model comprises of the three important clinical actions [20]:

(1) Ensuring that patients have the right *information (Knowledge)* and know how to adhere – including listening to patients' concerns, encouraging their participation and partnership in decision-making, building trust and empathy, and enhancing recall;

(2) Helping patients believe in their treatment and become *motivated* to commit to it – that is, addressing the cognitive, social, cultural normative and contextual factors that affect patients' beliefs, attitudes and motivation; and

(3) Assisting patients to overcome practical barriers to treatment adherence and develop a workable strategy for long-term disease management – including assessing and enhancing patients' social support, identifying and treating their depression and helping patients overcome cost-related treatment barriers.[20].

10.1. Knowledge regarding Antiretroviral treatment

The knowledge about HIV and AIDS and the benefits of ART are regarded as crucial for accepting the offer to get tested. Therefore, efforts should be made to intensify the dissemination of HIV and AIDS information and to fight stigma and discrimination in society. Since cultural background plays an important role in the individual response to HIV-related stigma, counseling and health education of patients should be adapted to cultural characteristics [21]. In addition, the study that was conducted in the Eastern Cape and recommended that an inaccuracy of the ART programme should be addressed; this should include improving knowledge translation during training of ART programme staff, ensuring the implementation of established data verification policies and procedures, rethinking the design of the programme to reduce the burden on health facilities and personnel, and standardizing information management procedures amongst the various governmental and non-governmental stakeholders. Knowledge is referred to as the facts known about the treatment, feelings or experiences by a person or group of people, the state of knowing, awareness, consciousness, or familiarity gained by experience or learning specific information about the subject [22].

A study conducted in Nigeria looked into PLHIVs knowledge about ARVs; they found out that HIV/AIDS knowledge was remarkably high. In addition, it was found that knowledge of ARV drug combinations, the appropriate time to start ARV, the benefits of taking ARV regularly and the possible results of not adhering to one's ARV medication was high among all the participants [23]. Furthermore, scores achieved by participants on knowledge about HIV, including the cause, mode of transmission and progression of the disease, were high, with an average score of 86%. In addition, the majority of patients were aware that taking ART could have side effects and knew that missing doses could lead to disease progression. In these studies it emerged that there was a need to reinforce educational messages that ART does not cure HIV and AIDS and that missing doses could cause drug resistance and lead to the progression of the disease. Whether or not good HIV and ART knowledge among these patients translates into good adherence needs further evaluation [24].

The patients' knowledge of ART is crucial in this study. It is the assertion of this thesis that if people living with HIV and AIDS were given information about the benefits and the side effects of ART and its impact on their wellbeing, the programme would have many more people on the treatment, if all systems were in place. It is also relevant to say that adherence would be less of a problem if people were given the relevant information and the support systems mentioned above were in place.

10.2. Attitudes to Antiretroviral treatment

The concept "attitude" is defined as a stable predisposition, a general and enduring positive or negative feeling about some person, object or issue [25]. In addition, attitudes originate from human cognition and are closely linked and influenced by perceptions. Prejudice and stigmatization refer to "a specific attitude which is a combination of hostile feelings, negative emotions and hostile behaviour towards others". Furthermore, an attitude is also defined as 'feelings of emotions and beliefs which influence the determination of behavior towards objects, persons or the environment"[26]. Furthermore, people's attitudes are made up of the cognitive - the knowledge and information they possess - and the affective - their feelings and emotions and evaluation of what is important.

Many personal attributes, such as commitment, positive self-esteem, motivation, ability to deal with stress and adaptability, have been used in research to explore and describe HIV and AIDS-related attitudes towards people living with HIV (PLHIV), and ART. Attitudes also include stigma and discrimination towards these people and towards ART, perceptions about ART, such as suggestions that is poisonous and not good for human consumption and that ART kills people. These perceptions lead to patients not taking the medication correctly, which ultimately leads to their resistance to the treatment and possibly dying.

10.3. Experiences of people living with HIV on Antiretroviral treatment

Knowledge gained from experience forms an essential aid to our understanding and activities in our everyday life. The experiences of PLHIV can be both negative and positive and this invariably affects their treatment process [27]. However, *"experience results in knowledge and understanding gained either individually or as a group or society through day-to-day living [28].*

The most immediate form of experience is personal experience, the body of knowledge gained individually through encountering situations and events in life". Patients living with HIV and AIDS experience a significant improvement in their health with fewer or no opportunistic infections; most patients regain their appetite and gain weight and experience increased energy levels.

A study was conducted that looked into the experiences of patients in ART programmes in KwaZulu-Natal. The results of the study indicate that many patients experienced financial problems which mean they encountered problems in obtaining appropriate food and paying for transportation to the nearest facility to collect their medication [28]. A three-country study was conducted in Uganda, Tanzania and Botswana, according to their study patients struggled with transport and user fees, long waiting times, lack of food, side effects from the medication, stigma and poor counseling[29]. Another study also found that scarcity of resources was a constant problem for adherence, and that patients had to beg, borrow or otherwise struggle to find funds for transport to obtain their monthly medication [30].

11. DISCUSSION OF THE FINDINGS
11.1. Introduction

The previous chapter presented all the data and findings of the study. In this chapter the researcher discusses a summary of the findings, conclusions and recommendations for both health authorities and for further research opportunities. These are discussed in relation to the objectives of the study as set out at the beginning. The researcher also outlines the identified strength and weaknesses of the study.

11.2. Sumary of Findings According to the Objectives

The main aims of the study were to investigate knowledge, attitudes and experiences of people living with HIV who are on ART at a public health clinic in Limpopo.

11.2.1. Objective 1: Knowledge of People Living with HIV Towards Antiretroviral Treatment

The first objective of the study was to investigate the knowledge of patients on ART the findings showed that the patients know ART, what it does in the human body, even though all five (100%) were unable to correctly pronounce the names of the ARVs. This is also supported by the information, motivation and behavior model which suggest that personal, behavioral and environmental factors largely determine one's actions[24]. Having a good knowledge and understanding of the benefits the patients can derive from adhering to ART may encourage the patients to take their treatment as required. All five of the participants interviewed (100%) shared positive outcomes and experiences while taking ART, including an improvement in physical, social and emotional wellbeing as well as greater optimism about the present and the future. This knowledge is crucial for patients to appreciate the importance of the ART and the required adherence for it to work optimally and produce positive outcomes. Although participants raised concerns of possible side-effects of medication, all of them (100%) mentioned that being on ART has enabled them to continue to care for their families and children and has been a great benefit. All indicated that they will never stop taking the treatment.

11.2.2. Objective 2: Attitudes of People Living with HIV Regarding Antiretroviral Treatment

All five of them (100%) reported feeling much better after taking the treatment and yielded better results. Participant said they trusted the nurses and felt that they were listened to, respected and given a chance to ask questions. Attitudes originate from human cognition and are closely linked and influenced by perceptions [25]. People's attitudes, change of behavior and optimal adherence depend on the knowledge, information, feelings and emotions they possess and this is supported by theoretical model used in this study, which indicates that inaccurate information plays an important role in negatively affecting adherence [31]. The IMB model of adherence, medication adherence is determined by the extent to which an individual is informed about his/her regimen, is motivated to adhere, and possesses the necessary behavioral skills to adhere in a variety of situations[32]. Furthermore, adherence information includes accurate knowledge about the regimen, potential side effects and drug interactions. In addition, adherence motivation is a function of personal and social motivation to adhere and personal motivation to adhere to regimen reflects an individual's attitudes about adherence and is based on one's beliefs that medication is helpful and not taking medication as prescribed would have undesirable consequences. However, having accurate knowledge or information about the treatment, the motivation and skills necessary to change the behaviour, is not a green light to optimal adherence but there are still factors such as disclosure of the status, the beliefs, experiences and the family and community support system, access to the health facility, reliable transport system and money can have an effect on whether the patient adheres to his or her treatment. The personal attributes such as positive self-esteem, commitment, ability to deal with stress and motivation are important in optimal adherence. In this study, all the participants have benefited from ART in a variety of ways, such as enhancing quality of life and fulfilling family obligations. All participants reported that they are happy about the programme, about the staff in the facility and about ART. However, challenges are still there and need the ART programme to address them in order to strengthen adherence and treatment outcomes.

11.2.3. Objective 3: Experiences of People Living With HIV Towards Antiretroviral Treatment

This research has revealed a numbers of experiences of people living with HIV and AIDS such as good knowledge of ART, positive attitudes towards ART and some concerns about the ART programme. The experience results in knowledge and understanding gained either individually or as a group or society through day-to-day living [33]. The most immediate form of experience reported by all participants was a personal experience, the body of knowledge gained individually through encountering situations and events in this HIV/AIDS journey of life. Challenges such as a lack of knowledge by employers, poverty and unemployment were reported as some of the barriers to optimal adherence. The researcher observed during clinic visits, that written information and materials about adherence and treatment guidelines and protocols to reinforce adherence are available in the clinic. The participants interviewed were generally happy with the outcomes of treatment. Some participants complained about side-effects early during the treatment and the demanding nature of ARV regimens. Almost all participants experienced problems during the early days of the treatment and there were advised to stick to treatment.

11.2.4. Objective 4: Economic Factors that Support People Living with HIV

Social and economic factors may combine to yield poor adherence outcomes in South Africa. In addition, many patients studied experienced financial constraints for food and transportation to the nearest facility to collect medication, long waiting times, poverty and hunger, lack social support, side effects and lack of appropriate counseling. All these factors undermine the adherence to antiretroviral treatment[34]. It is crucial to note that in this study three (60 %) of the participants reported having no problems adhering to their treatment whilst two (40%) agreed and admitted having stopped ART for more than a month prior for these interviews which is in essence non-adherence to treatment as it was prematurely stopped. The findings show that there is generally poor adherence to treatment regimes in this study. A study in Tanzania, Uganda and Botswana concludes that costs of food and transport to and from the clinic serve as a deterrent to ART optimal adherence [29]. Transport costs and money for food were reported to be a burden for almost all respondents and a treatment-related increase in appetite posed an additional challenge especially because most of the respondents are not employed and depend on the government grant and "piece jobs". However, the government provides some nutritional support if needed in the form of nutritional supplements provided by the dieticians in the clinic and also a grant in the form of monetary value on a monthly basis depending on the status of the patients.

12. CONCLUSION

The aim of this study was to investigate the knowledge, attitudes and experiences of people living with HIV and on ART at the Witpoort Hospital, Limpopo Province. It is envisaged that the findings of this study will help the health care professionals and the Provincial Department of Health to develop intervention strategies and programmes that will help in identifying those patients at risk of non-adhering to treatment and those that need support for optimal adherence. The most commonly reported experiences on ART in this study were inability to take treatment at work, being just too lazy to go to clinic for follow-up visits and forgetting to take the treatment. It also emerged that a lack of HIV and AIDS knowledge of the employers and colleagues contributed to some participants not adhering to their treatment.

13. REFERENCES

1. Thomas, E.(2014). South Africa was oncenotorious for apartheid. Emerging Johannesburg. Routledge. P185
2. Rouzier, V, Farmer, P.E, and Pape, W. (2014). Factors impacting the provision of Antiretroviral Therapy to people living with HIV. The view from Haiti. Antivir. Therapy. 19(3), 91-104
3. Cummings, B., Gutin, S.A. and Jaiantilal, P. (2014). The Role of Social Support Among People Living with HIV in Rural Mozambique. *AIDS Patient Care and STDs*, 602-612.
4. Peltzer, K., Ramlagan, S., Jones, D., Weiss, S. M., Fomundam, H. and Chanetsa, L. (2012). Efficacy of a lay health worker led group antiretroviral medication adherence training among non-adherent HIV-positive patients in KwaZulu-Natal, South Africa: Results from a randomized trial. SaharaJ: *Journal of Social Aspects of HIV/AIDS*, 9(4), 218-226. doi: 10.1080/17290376.2012.745640
5. Dunbar-Jacob, J., Schenk, E. and McCall, M. (2012). 12 Patient Adherence to Treatment Regimen. *Handbook of Health Psychology*, Psychology Press, 271.
6. Dewing, S., Mathews, C. and Lurie M. (2015). Predictors of poor adherence among people on antiretroviral treatment in Cape Town, South Africa: a case-control study. *AIDS Care*, 342-349.
7. Gioia, D.A., Corley, K.G. and Hamilton, A.L. (2013). Seeking qualitative rigor in inductive research notes on the Gioia methodology. O*rganisational Research Methods*, 16(1). 15-31.
8. Perez, A., Holt, N., Gokiert, R., Chanoine, J.P., Legault, L., Morrison, K., Sharma A. and Ball, G. (2015). Why don't families initiate treatment? A qualitative multicentre study investigating parents' reasons for declining paediatric weight management. *Paediatrics & Child Health*, 20(4) 179-84
9. Creswell, J.W. (2013). Research design: Qualitative, quantitative, and mixed methods approaches. Thousand Oaks. CA:Sage publications.
10. Hulley, S.B., Cummings, S.R. and Browner, W.S. (2013). *Designing clinical research*. Lippincott Williams & Wilkins.
11. Denscombe, M. (2014). *The good research guide: for small-scale social research projects*. UK: McGraw-Hill Education
12. Robinson, O.C. (2014). Sampling in interview-based qualitative research: A theoretical and practical guide, *Qualitative Research in Psychology*, 11(1). 25-41.
13. Sandelowski, M. (1995). Focus on Qualitative Methods. Sample Size in Qualitative Research. *Research in Nursing and Health* 18:179-183.
14. Collins, K.M.T., Onwuegbuzie, A.J. and Jiao, Q.G. (2006). Prevalence of mixed methods sampling designs in social science research. Evaluation and Research in Education 19(2): 83-101
15. Corbin, J. and Strauss A. (2014). Basics of qualitative research: Techniques and procedures for developing grounded theory. Thousand Oaks. CA: Sage publications.
16. Irvine, A., Drew, P. and Sainsburry, R. (2013). Am I not answering your questions properly? Clarification, adequacy and responsiveness in semi-structured telephone and face-to-face interviews, *Qualitative Research*, 13(1). 87-102.
17. Mertens, D.M. (1998). Research methods in education and psychology: Integrating diversity with qualitative and quantitative approaches. London. Sage Publications.
18. Babbie, E.R. (2010). T*he practice of social research*. Belmont: Wadsworth, Cengage Learning.

19. Henn, M., Weinstein, M. and Foard, N. (2006). *A Short Introduction to Social Research*. London: Sage Publications.
20. DiMatteo, M., Haskard-Zolnierek, K.B., and Martin, L. (2012). Improving patient adherence: a three-factor model to guide practice. *Health Psychology Review*,74-91.
21. Seeling, S., Mavhunga F. and Thoma, A.B. (2014). Barriers to access to antiretroviral treatment for HIV-positive tuberculosis patients in Windhoek, Namibia. *International Journal of Mycobacteriology*, 3(4). 268-275.
22. Kaposhi, B.M., Moqoqi, N. and Schoopflocher, P. (2015). Evaluation of antiretroviral treatment programme monitoring in Eastern Cape, South Africa. *Health Policy and Planning*, 30(5). 547-554.
23. Weiser, S.D., Tuller, D.M. and Frongillo, E.A. (2010). Food insecurity as a barrier to sustained antiretroviral therapy in Uganda. PLoS one. 5(4). 1.
24. Munthli, A., Mvula, P.M. and Maluwa-Banda, D. (2014). Knowledge, attitudes and practices about HIV testing and counselling among adolescent girls in some selected secondary schools in Malawi, *African Journal of Reproductive Health*, 17(4). 60-68.
25. Sellam, D. and Flower, F.L. (2014). A study on stigma towards people living with HIV/AIDS in perambalur district, *Star. Soc. Work.* 2(5). 98.
26. Beaulieu, M., Andrien, A. and Potvin, L. (2014). Stigmatizing attitudes towards people living with HIV/AIDS: validation of a measurement scale. *BMC Public Health*, 1246.
27. French, H., Greef M. and Watson, M. (2015). HIV stigma and disclosure experiences of people living with HIV in an urban and a rural setting. *AIDS Care*, 27(8), 1-5.
28. Nsanzimana, S., Prabhu, K. and McDermott, H. (2015). Improving health outcomes through concurrent HIV program scale-up and health system development in Rwanda: 20 years of experience. *BMC medicine*, 13(1). 216.
29. Hardon, A.P., Akurut, D, Comoro, C., and Ekezie, C. (2007). Hunger, waiting time and transport costs: Time to confront challenges to ART adherence in Africa. AIDS care 19(5). 658-665
30. Ware, N.C. (2009). Explaining adherence success in Sub-Saharan Africa: An ethnographic study: PLoS Med 6(1).
31. Fisher, J. and Amico, K.R. (2008). The information, motivation, and behavioral skills model of ART adherence to Antiretroviral Therapy, Health Psychology, 25(4).
32. Mayberry, L.S. and Osborn, C. (2014). Empirical validation of Information, Motivation and Behaioural Skills Model of Diabetes Medication Adherence: A Framework for Intervention. Diabetes Care (37). 1246-7263.
33. Yoder, P., Mkhize, S.P. and Nzimande, S. (2009). *Patient Experiences in Antiretroviral Therapy Programmes in KwaZulu-Natal, South Africa*. Durban, South Africa: Health Systems Trust and Calverton, Maryland, USA: Macro International Inc.
34. Kagee, A. (2006). Adherence to antiretroviral treatment in the context of national rollout in South Africa: Defining a research agenda for psychology. *South African Journal of Psychology* 38(2):413-428.

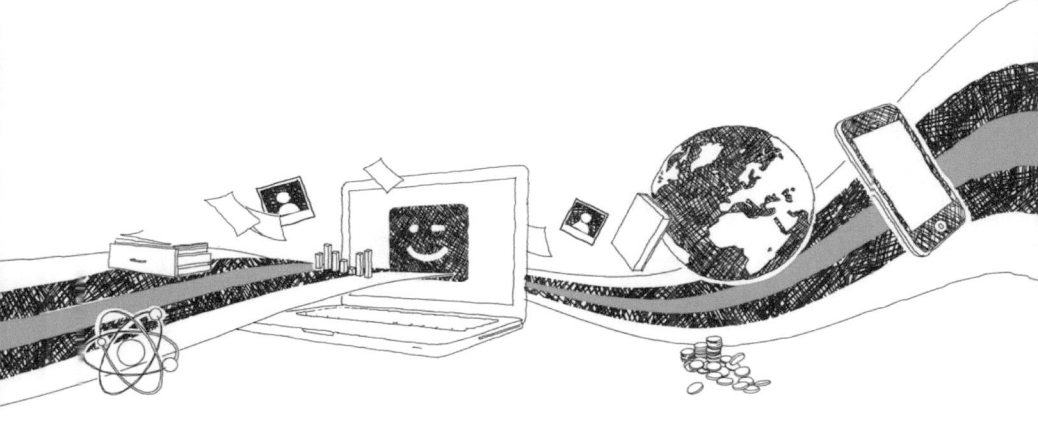